Your B
Week For Week

Introduction

I'd like to thank you for downloading the book, *"Your Baby Guide Week For Week"*.

This book gives you a comprehensive understanding of how your baby is developing week for week as well as what it is you should do to ensure you have a healthy and successful pregnancy.

Are you planning to get pregnant, just missed your periods and are suspecting that you could be pregnant or have already confirmed that you are pregnant? If either of these is true, congratulations-you are about to become a mother.

But while this is definitely good news, you probably are worried; worried about whether you will carry the baby to full term, worried about the morning sickness, worried about the health of the baby that you are carrying and such. So what is it you can do to minimize your level of worry? Simple; you equip yourself with as much knowledge about pregnancy as possible so that you can approach it with all the confidence you need.

This book provides all that i.e. knowledge to take you throughout your pregnancy from the 1st week to the day you get to hold your bundle of joy in your arms. It breaks down your term into weeks so you can learn how your baby is developing, how to take care of it while in the womb, the changes taking place in your body throughout the pregnancy and such.

After reading the book, you can bet that you will be better equipped to deal with anything that comes up during the pregnancy from a point of knowledge as opposed to a point of fear. While your doctor/OB may give you much of the information, having lots of knowledge about pregnancy will provide a good enough foundation for your discussions with your OB or doctor even if you are a first time mom.

Thanks again for downloading this book. I hope you enjoy it!

information is without contract or any type of guarantee assurance.

The trademarks that are used are without any consent, and the publication of the trademark is without permission or backing by the trademark owner. All trademarks and brands within this book are for clarifying purposes only and are the owned by the owners themselves, not affiliated with this document.

Table of Contents

Before we can start highlighting the changes happening to you and the baby as well as what it is you should to do increase your chances of a safe and healthy pregnancy, let's learn some basics about pregnancy first.

Let's Get Some Facts Right First

Pregnancy can last between 38-42 weeks with 40 weeks being the average. However, since doctors cannot with absolute certainty tell when an egg is fertilized (i.e. conception takes place) given that the day when an egg is released is not standard and the fact that sperms can last for up to a week and still be viable, doctors usually use an estimate of 40 weeks from the first day of the last menstruation period to determine the expected due date.

This means that before you actually become pregnant; your baby is usually estimated to be 1-2 weeks old! Interestingly, it takes a further 6 or more weeks to confirm that you are pregnant! As you probably know, the pregnancy duration (often referred to as 'term') is grouped into 3 months trimesters in which various changes take place both in your body and your baby's body. Within this duration, you need to be physically and emotionally prepared to deal with pregnancy signs and symptoms. Furthermore, you should learn what to eat or avoid, healthcare to seek for, exercising tips and how the baby daddy can be of help. This book offers guidelines on how to carry on with your pregnancy especially if you're a first time mom. Let's start right away from your first trimester of pregnancy:

The First Trimester

Week 1 & Week 2

At this point, you are not really pregnant since no conception has taken place. That's why we've combined the first 2 weeks to show you what's happening to your body before you are actually pregnant.

In the first week of pregnancy, you may probably have cramps where your uterus sheds off last month's unfertilized egg (menstruation) marking the start of your next cycle. At this time, your body prepares itself for ovulation, which is likely to take place 11-19 days after the first day of your last menstruation. The preparation in this case entails priming the next egg for maturity so that it can be released to the fallopian tube. All this happens in a carefully coordinated and orchestrated biological clock run by hormones. The hormone responsible for stimulating the eggs (contained in follicles) to mature is the follicle-stimulating hormone (FSH). As the follicles mature, they start producing estrogen and progesterone hormones, which in turn help initiate the process of repairing and thickening the walls of your uterus. When the time is right, estrogen triggers the luteinizing hormone (LH) to make the most mature follicle (which contains the maturing egg) to burst through the ovarian wall 24-36 hours after the LH surge (this takes place about 12-14 days into the cycle). This is what's referred to as ovulation. From then on, your body is ready to meet a sperm cell for fusion.

As the released ovum is heading to the uterus, estrogen hormone triggers the uterine wall to thicken and to form blood rich lining of tissue. As a result, you may feel one-sided pain, breast soreness, heavy boobs, mild cramping and PMS. It's also a common thing to detect odors as ovulation causes the body to become sensitive to smells. Progesterone (I mentioned it earlier) helps a fertilized ovum get implanted into your uterus if conception takes place.

So what dietary and health measures should you be taking during the first 2 weeks even if you are not actually pregnant?

Healthcare and Dieting

If you are already intending to become pregnant, this is the time to taking folic acid supplements to help prevent possible pregnancy complications. Lack of minerals such as iron can lead to a serious condition that affects the nervous system of your baby, a condition referred to as *spina bifida*. Furthermore, you should stop drinking alcohol or smoking cigarettes and other drugs as these too could affect your baby negatively.

Week 3

The actual conception takes place this week where a single sperm cell fuses with the ovum already released from the ovaries after ovulation. Fertilization takes place in your fallopian tube 45 minutes to 7 days after sexual activity. The fastest swimmers can get to the fallopian tube within 45 minutes after intercourse although 12 hours is the average but if they don't find an egg, they can wait for up to 7 days, which means if you were to ovulate within the 7 days, you could still conceive. The mature ova can only last for about 24 hours after which it loses its viability if it is not fertilized within this window. If the conditions for fertilization are met and the respective cells, ova and sperm, are present, fusion takes place.

Note: if you don't conceive, the ovaries stop producing more estrogen and progesterone, the two hormones, which are essential for sustaining a pregnancy. As the presence of the two hormones facilitates the thickening of the lining of the uterus, the decline of these results to shedding of the thickening (what happens during your period) along with the unfertilized egg.

The fusion between the sperm and the ovum forms a zygote, and the fertilized egg forms a barrier to inhibit entry of other sperms. From a single cell, the zygote undergoes cell division within a few hours to form two cells, and then four and the cycle of division continues. All this takes place as the zygote moves down the fallopian tubes towards the uterus (this takes a few days).

At some point (after about 4-6 days), 100 multiple identical cells referred to as blastocyst are formed, ready to be implanted on the uterus (see below). Although being a microscopic ball of cells, soon, some of these cells will constitute the embryo and others will form the placenta. As I stated, the blastocyst stage of the embryo starts at around 4-6 days after fertilization. In this case, fluid starts filling inside the embryo resulting to the formation of a fairly small cavity. On the other hand, the outer cells start creating a wall while the inner cells start forming a ball (this is what will become the baby!). You can learn more about the fertilization and implantation process here.

Note: As implantation happens, you should start noting some spotting at the vulva as a result of the blastocyst burrowing into your blood-rich uterine lining.

Soon after fertilization, the baby starts to develop all the features of a human being although not visible by the human eye. The external part of the blastocyst starts to develop into the placenta as the internal part starts forming the embryo. Unknown to you, the sex of the unborn child is already determined as a result of cells referred to as chromosomes. A fertilized egg has 46 chromosomal cells, 23 cells from your body usually abbreviated as XX; and the remaining 23 cells from the dad abbreviated as XY. Since your cells are XX, you can only contribute X chromosome but the dad can contribute either X or Y chromosome. In case the sperm carries the Y chromosome, the baby would be a boy, as the fusion will produce XY cells found in men. On the other hand, if the sperm carries X chromosome, you'll get a girl child as females carry XX chromosomal combination. You can learn more about the science of conception here. Within the first 24 hours, the zygote changes from being a zygote to an embryo (see more here).

If you got pregnant (which you may not know by now though), the first thing you need to do is think about your health- your baby depends on it.

Healthcare and Dieting

The first healthcare step to take is to visit a dentist for teeth check as most pregnant mums experience bleeding gums. The condition is caused by increased blood supply to most body organs and dental services can help curb possible complications. Also, ensure that you follow a proper diet as well.

Week 4

What's happening to the baby?

The new-formed embryo begins to develop within the uterine lining of your womb, as the outer cells connect to your blood system. Being less than 3mm in length, the embryonic form starts to change from two to three layers of cells. With the placenta bringing in nutrients and carrying away waste products, the baby also develops an amniotic sac. This sac is a protection barrier against shock and other dangers and is meant to remain until delivery.

At this point, the embryo divides into 3 layers, with the outer layer, also called ectoderm, developing into the skin, hair, eyes and the brain. The mesoderm or the middle layer develops into kidneys, heart, bones, muscles and sex organs. The inner layer referred to as endoderm develops into the liver, lungs and various digestive organs. For now, the embryo is attached to tiny yolk sac that facilitates nourishment before the placenta fully develops to a point of becoming fully functional. The placental cells are growing into the womb to facilitate rich supply of blood, nutrients and oxygen.

As all this happens, your body is also changing.

Your body changes

At this juncture, you may not feel major signs of pregnancy despite occasional fatigue and nausea as your body continues secreting hormones to support baby growth. Other possible signs may include mood swings, bloating and menstrual cramps that could be accompanied with implantation bleeding. As the embryo gets implanted on the uterine lining, you might feel a little pressure at your abdomen. In case you feel your breasts are getting tender and even a little sore, it's because your mammary glands are triggered to start maturing.

Week 5

Let's start with how the baby is changing

With the baby being shielded by protective membranes and joined to the yolks sac, major changes start to take place. For instance, the inner, middle and outer layers of the embryo begin to develop into various organs among them the spinal cord, the heart, blood vessels and the brain. At first, a hollow tube referred to as neural tube forms from the ectoderm and eventually develops into the brain and spinal cord. The tube-like structure also has a bulge at the center, which develops to form the heart; and then separates into 4 chambers to begin pumping blood.

What about your body?

Body changes

By now, you might not be sure whether you are pregnant or not but the situation of a missed period should suggest "something". This is the time to take a pregnancy test to confirm it by simply determining the levels of <u>hCG (Human chorionic gonadotropin) hormone</u> in urine. Apart from the persistent fatigue, you're also likely to experience nausea and frequent urination. Due to the increase in the blood volume that could hit over 150 percent, a surplus liquid is secreted and eventually gets into the bladder; triggering frequent urination. Another thing is that the growing uterus can push the bladder down and disrupt storage of urine.

Week 6

If this is your 6th week of pregnancy (according to the doctors), you are actually 4 weeks pregnant! Here is what's happening to the baby.

During this week, the ¼-inch long embryo curves into a tail-like structure that resembles a tadpole. The arms and legs, which are starting to become visible (very tiny though) now resemble stubs as they protrude from the body. At the sides of the head, the embryo develops little dimples, which grow into ears and nostrils, and a thickening appears at the face to represent the eyes. As circulation of blood is now possible through the umbilical cord, the lungs, liver, pancreases and intestines continue to develop. Arms and legs also begin to form thick webbing between developing fingers or toes, and the skin at this point is translucent without pigmentation.

So what's happening to your body as all the above takes place?

Your body changes

Although the blood volume has already increased significantly, you're more likely to feel dizzy and exhausted due to your blood dropping in pressure. Another thing is that hormones such as progesterone have surged and this could worsen symptoms of morning sickness. However, although these signs could be troublesome and heart breaking, medics are of the view that such pregnancy symptoms show you're less likely to develop miscarriage.

Week 7

The embryo is now about 10-13mm long but appears a little strange since the head is twice bigger than other body parts. The larger forehead is due to the rapid development of the brain and is meant to remain that way until week 36. This week, your baby's inner ears start to develop, and the limb buds forms a cartilage that develops to form the legs or arms bones. The arm buds also elongate and hands begin to be formed as the nerve cells multiply to constitute the nervous system. Likewise, the leg buds separate into the foot, knee and leg segments.

The embryo's forehead now develops facial features such as mouth and tongue, and eyes (tissues such as lenses and retina get joined together into eyes). However, the eyelid is folding and can partially cover the eyes, which remain closed until week 26. Organs such as kidneys start to function and start to excrete urine from the embryo's digestive system into the amniotic fluid. Moreover, the embryo swallows the amniotic fluid, which is digested into urine and eventually excreted through your bladder. On the other hand, the liver begins to produce red blood cells, which determine the specific blood type your baby has.

As all this takes place, your body is also changing.

Your body changes

The main body change you'd note is the breast enlargement that is caused by increased blood supply and continuous fat storage under them. In some women, it's likely that the dark area of the nipple (areola) may grow in size and become darker. Other symptoms such as fatigue and morning sickness are likely to persist; and you might also notice considerable reduction in your waistline. Moreover, although you might not realize it, your cervix mucus plug also gets thick to help seal the uterus up until you give birth.

Week 8

Almost 2 months down the line, the embryo has grown big enough to now become a fetus, or what can be referred to an "offspring". Now weighing 2-3 grams and being slightly over ½ inch long, the fetus loses the embryonic tail. The fetus is still enclosed in the amniotic sac inside the uterus, and the placenta now develops blood vessels or villi that attach placenta to the womb. This week, the legs lengthen to form a bone-like cartilage, though distinct parts of the legs aren't formed yet.

Other bones such as the joints and elbows begin to harden and take shape in what can be referred to as ossification. The webbed feet and hands also begin to elongate and separate into fingers; and by now, the nose, ears, jaw-line and mouth parts are becoming more visible. Unknown to you, the fetus can start to make slight movements.

Your body is also preparing for motherhood by having different changes.

Your body changes

As the fetus continues to develop, you might feel sharp pain at the sides of the pelvis caused by the uterus forcing down the ligaments that hold it in place. Due to increase in the estrogen and hCG hormone, morning sickness symptoms may continue to persist. Furthermore, the muscles of the digestive tract may relax and make digestion ineffective as the progesterone level surges and the uterine wall muscles stretch further. You might also note a pink discharge from your cervix but this is a normal thing; otherwise see a doctor if the discharge is heavy, clotted or bright red.

Note: Bleeding or spotting during pregnancy especially for the first 13 weeks or so is okay unless bleeding becomes heavy.

To take care of the growing baby (now fetus), you will need to take care of your body. Let's take a look at some things you ought to do:

Healthcare and Dieting

It's advisable to eat lightly especially if you have digestive problems among them heartburn. Other symptoms such as vomiting and nausea should disappear by week 14 so don't be afraid of eating. If losing appetite, why not eat a fruit? Fruits are rich in vitamins and nutrients and can be a great alternative to eating veggies. Choose fruits such as dried apricots, cantaloupe, red apple and deeply hued melons.

Week 9

At this point, the basic structure of the eyes has been formed and the baby is around ¾ inch long. However, the eyelids shut or fuse together, where they will reopen during the 27th week of pregnancy. As the arms and fingers have developed bones, the hands can now touch the face. The intestines now begin to move away from the umbilical cord and into the abdomen as the body grows in size. The sex organs referred to as gonads also develop into testes for boys and ovaries for girls; but the gender may not be distinguishable yet. You have to wait for an <u>ultrasound scan</u> in your second trimester.

So what happens to your body during this week?

Your body changes

The level of nausea should be at its peak now but starting next week, you should feel better as the hormonal levels stabilize. The uterus size has doubled and is the size of a tennis ball; and the area below your navel has become firmer. To some women, the skin and hair complexion can change, and might feel limp and greasy due to surging hormonal levels. Taking walks can help you feel better.

What about diet and healthcare; what should you do this week?

Healthcare and Dieting

It's advisable that you get your first antenatal appointment also known as <u>booking appointment</u> for your blood sample routine checks during this week. Have your doctor or midwife conduct <u>various tests</u> to evaluate how your pregnancy is developing.

Week 10

Most bones and joints are well developed such as the ankles, shoulders, knees, wrists and elbows alongside the toes, feet, hands and fingers. Likewise, external ears become evident on the side of the baby's head, as ear canals are formed inside the head. The heart, the kidney or the lungs can function on their own, and now the heart is beating 180 times per minute, about twice or thrice your heart beat. Looking at the baby's face, a medical expert can observe the upper lip and two small nostrils. These changes happen as the jawbones develop to incorporate the future milk teeth. At 1½ inches length, your baby may also be making small jerky movements notable on the ultrasound scan.

And as your baby makes these milestones, you too are changing.

Your body changes

Morning sickness symptoms start to reduce as the hormonal level subsides. However, you might notice prominent veins at major areas such as legs, breasts and tummy caused by increased blood supply to these areas. The breasts also increase in size to 1 or 2 bra cup sizes as progesterone hormone stimulates milk glands to develop. The nipples also expand, become darker and erect as the milk ducts develop.

What about diet-should you be eating for two?

Healthcare and Dieting

Worried about too much weight? Whatever the case, don't diet during pregnancy, as most of the weight will come off soon after delivery. Ensure that you consume nutritious foods in sufficient quantities to counter additional weight gain as the baby continues to grow. Remember to attend screening for any chromosomal defects among them the Down syndrome.

Week 11

At 2 inches, the baby's head will appear to constitute about a third of its full length. Gradually, the fetus' body starts straightening and its fingernails form, and eventually, the fingers and toes completely separate. However, the skin still remains transparent. Moreover, the fetus is surrounded by amniotic fluid, which it's learning to swallow. It can still stretch, sigh a little, suck its thumb and move its head, and soon the baby's size will double in size. Sex organs such as testis and ovaries are under development.

While all this is taking place, you too are changing.

Your Body Changes

As you get towards the second trimester, a dark vertical pigment can appear on your belly referred to as linea nigra. Furthermore, it's likely for the abdomen to protrude and you feel bloated as the digestion process slows down. This happens because the progesterone hormone (which is high during this time) relaxes your gastrointestinal tract to enable nutrients to be assimilated into the blood; this can make you uncomfortable.

During this week, you will need to be careful with your health as well.

Healthcare and Dieting

The key to good health is to attend prenatal testing as these tests can alleviate fears about the condition of your unborn baby. You should also drink more water to facilitate increased production of sweat, blood, amniotic fluid and other bodily fluids. Thus, drink ample water and milk, and carry un-carbonated beverages with you to replenish your body fluids.

Week 12

At the end of the first trimester, the fetus weighs half-an-ounce, and measures about 2½ inches long. By now, most organs are fully formed among them the muscles, organs, bones and limbs, and the sex organs can almost depict the gender of your baby. So far, the baby's skeleton is composed of cartilage, a special tissue that will soon develop into a hard bone. The vocal cords and the brain tissue continue to mature and the nerve cells undergo rapid cell division.

The fetus has now mastered natural movements such as clenching and opening the fists, bending the arms and twisting of the elbows. These movements now become more frequent as the brain muscle develops and starts sending brain signals. Other facial features such as lips and eyebrows now come into focus.

While your body is having milestones, you too have your own milestones:

Your body changes

This week, the uterus should shift up and forward to help relieve the pressure at your bladder and possibly reduce your frequent urination. You might also feel less tired amid slight headaches as the blood volume in your body increases.

Healthcare and Dieting

To sustain the pregnancy, ensure that you eat foods high in fiber and drink water to keep the intestinal tract functional. And since you might be in such a good mood, it's the high time to exercise with your partner; for instance you can have a walk to the park while holding hands.

Pregnancy Tips For The First Trimester

1. Ensure That You Budget For Your Pregnancy

Even for the unplanned pregnancy, early planning will save you from future financial problems. If you don't have any insurance cover catering for delivery costs, you should probably start saving now to ensure that you have enough money for all possible costs.

2. Ensure That You Eat Right

Right from your first stages of early pregnancy, you need to start eating right; make a good diet plan to follow to help you with the development of the baby. Eat more proteins and nutrients, especially folate, zinc, iron and iodine; but basically adopt variety of foods including all the five food groups. This is because your nutrient requirements during pregnancy increase to maintain your health and support the developing baby. To get necessary nutrients, eat these minerals from various foods:

- *Folate and folic acid*

Folate is a vitamin B that occurs naturally in green leafy vegetables, fruits such as citrus, bananas and berries, and legumes. Lack of enough folate in the early stages of pregnancy has been associated with increased risks of neural tube defects like spina bifida. On top of folate foods, include an additional 400 micrograms of folic acid per day, for the first part of the trimester.

- *Iron*

As your blood volume increases to meet the demands of your baby and the placenta, it's likely to become iron deficient. Thus, ensure to include iron-rich foods such as red meat, fish, pork and chicken as well as green leafy veggies, iron fortified cereals and legumes. To help your body absorb iron from plants, eat foods rich in vitamin C such as oranges and tomatoes.

- *Zinc*

You need zinc for normal growth and development of the brain, bones and various parts of the body. You can get it from a wide variety of foods such as fish, dairy and red meat, and plant sources to a lesser extent such as cereals, legumes and nuts.

- *Iodine*

Iodine is very important for the development of your baby's nervous system and brain. Moreover, your body's iodine requirements increase during pregnancy by 47% percent and a whopping 80% when you are breastfeeding. Valuable sources of iodine include seafood, fortified bread and dairy.

Avoid Foods Such As Raw Eggs During Pregnancy

It is possible to over indulge in certain foods especially when cravings start to develop. However, you need to be nutrition conscious. For instance, avoid the following:

- *Raw meat and eggs*

Avoid taking raw or undercooked eggs and meat, as well as pate, as these are potential hosts of bacteria that could cause harm to your baby. Also avoid raw seafood such as sushi or oyster that has not been frozen before preparing.

- *Sea foods*

Avoid swordfish, marlin or shark, as these fish are perilous sources of naturally occurring mercury. Tuna also has some mercury, so it is best to minimize its intake to less than 4 medium sized cans, or eat two fresh tuna steaks every week.

- *Cheeses*

Don't take cheeses that have a white and moldy rind like camembert and brie, as well as blue veined cheeses like Roquefort. All these might contain listeria, a form of bacteria that might be harmful to your baby.

- *Liver products*

Liver and liver products such as liver sausage and pate may contain unsafe levels of the retinol form of vitamin A whose consumption in excess can harm your baby.

- *Alcohol and caffeine*

When pregnant, stop or cut down on alcohol intake to one or two units of alcohol, at most twice a week. For caffeine, limit it to 200mg per day, equivalent to two mugs of instant coffee, or five cans of cola, or 4 cups of tea per day. Instead, drink decaffeinated colas and hot drinks.

That said; don't follow any dieting programs especially because some diets can render you deficient of folic acid, iron and other important minerals and vitamins. You can improve your diet if you are overweight by reducing foods rich in sugar (simple sugars) and unhealthy fat and doing some exercise.

4. Do Regular Exercises Often

Doing regular exercise such as walking can prepare you to get back to your normal weight after birth. However, avoid strenuous exercises such as yoga, scuba diving or contact sports where the baby bump may risk getting hit. Also, avoid activities that may affect your balance making you fall over, such as cycling or horse riding. To avoid damaging the joints, you should avoid jumping or running, which leaves walking as the most recommended exercise.

5. Have your partner support you

There are various things that your baby daddy can contribute to stress-free pregnancy such as:

-Taking you for prenatal appointment, where he can inquire about various tests and suggested exercising routine for you. Later, you can enjoy a meal together and discuss about the happenings of the appointment.

-Be kind to yourself when tormented by morning sickness, which tends to suppress sexual desires. Also, understand when hormones surge and turn you almost into a "sex maniac"!

-Continue to love yourself even after breast enlargement or uncontrollable weight gain that can mess your perfect figure.

-As you sing moody blues for your fetus, let the daddy hum along with you. Always give room for him to share his excitement, fears and expectations about your pregnancy.

-After coming home, your man can surprise you with a gift such as flowers, and should also give you a break when needed.

Second Semester

Week 13

The fetus has now entered the second semester of pregnancy, and may now weigh about 25 grams while measuring 3 inches long. One of the major changes taking place this week is the testes and ovaries becoming fully developed inside the body. Due to this new development, noticeable genitalia are beginning to form outside the fetus' body so an ultrasound scan can reveal the gender. Under ultrasound equipment, the fetus resembles a small baby, albeit extremely smaller; its eyes could be moving from the side of the head drawing closer towards each other. As the eyes respond, the fine hairs that constitute the eyebrows also come together.

Another great change that is taking place is the intestinal system of your baby becoming fully functional. This week, the abdomen develops fully to enable the intestines to relocate to the correct position. The fetus' liver can also secrete bile and the pancreas is able to produce insulin that would be helpful in controlling the level of sugar after childbirth. Although the head remains significantly soft, other bones continue to harden further; and the vocal cords begin to form.

Your body is also changing during this week.

Your body changes

This week, you'll be more energetic with less nausea, which should completely disappear by week 15. However, your taste and smell aversions could be persistent throughout the pregnancy although this shouldn't be a big bother.

Diet and exercise

Moreover, it is recommendable to start a new exercise now such as swimming, which can be paired with low-impact exercises like yoga preferably through specialized prenatal yoga class. When you work out in water, the abdominal muscles are both engaged and lengthened, as they're involved in keeping you balanced. That's not all; the buoyancy of water makes it easier for you to hold poses like <u>yoga's Warrior III (shown below)</u> that may not be possible to hold on land. At the end you get better toning benefit and you're able to do deeper stretches.

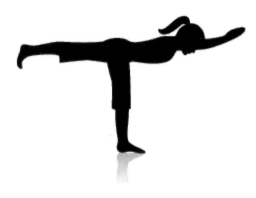

Week 14

Your fetus is about 85mm long, being the size of a clenched fist and has grown enough to be able to leap or stand up straight. These movements are facilitated by the full maturity of the neck, which now supports the head to stand straight. The fetus swallows little bits of amniotic fluid to its stomach and the kidneys help to remove the fluid as urine. The fetus may also be able to suck the thumb and may make more facial expressions such as squinting and frowning. At this stage, its body is covered with a downy coating of hair referred to as lanugo, which assists in keeping warm.

Your body changes

In this semester, your breasts are less as tender and the episodes of frequent urination or morning sickness will soon be forgotten. This semester, your uterus will rise out of the pelvic region and into the lower abdomen.

A few weeks to come, you should feel the top of the uterus if you press down right above the pelvic bone into the lower abdomen. The rapid uterine growth can trigger round ligament pain that occurs on both sides of the abdomen. As the uterus is supported by thick bands of ligaments, expansion of the uterus stretches the ligaments and triggers the sharp pain. The pain is evident when you change positions rapidly, when coughing or after you get up from a seat. To help reduce the pain, try putting the feet up and rest in a relaxed pose.

Week 15

Being about 4-5 inches long, the fetus can make noticeable body movements such as kicks characterized by occasional hiccups. Never mind as the developing being can hear sounds or noises from your breathing, digestive system, heartbeat and your voice. In other times, you can feel the occasional breathing, swallowing or sucking practices it makes while responding to various stimuli. Another major development that the fetus undergoes is response to light. Even though closed, the eyes become sensitive to light and may register bright light outside the tummy.

Your body changes

The pelvic area is likely to feel firm and heavy since your uterus is carrying almost a full cup of amniotic fluid. It's highly likely that you gain a few pounds henceforth due to the extra pounds from your fetus and the extra fluid and blood volume. Furthermore, the enlarging breasts, placenta and other fetus support systems contribute to weight gain. If necessary, you might consider undergoing an ultra-sound scan to check for any genetic defects.

Week 16

Weighing around 3-5 ounces, the fetus can utilize its own breathing system to either inhale or exhale surrounding amniotic fluid. Furthermore, its heart can now pump about 25 quarts of blood a day, and can clearly hear your voice or your partner's. In some cases, loud noises such as loud music, doorbell rings or dog barking can startle the fetus. At this time, the skin that has been transparent begins to gain a darker pigment, although the blood vessels are clearly visible. The lean skin may also start to accumulate fat deposits, which would later act as insulation for the baby after lanugo disappears.

Your body changes

Most pregnant moms are likely to experience stuffy noses or possible nose bleeds due to blood volume increase (blood volume could increase by up to 50%). Blood increase affects estrogen hormonal levels, which in turn cause the nasal membranes to swell. Although it is not advisable to use antihistamine nasal sprays, you can use nasal strips or saline sprays in cases where your congestion is uncomfortable. Dab some petroleum jelly under the nose to combat dryness brought about by nasal congestion, or use a humidifier instead. Apart from congestions, the blood volume may trigger the heart to work harder than usual but it's less likely to develop heart complications. The ligaments also stretch and this might make you feel pain and aches around the belly.

Week 17

The fetus weighs about 5 ounces, and its skeleton is made-up of rubbery cartilage meant to harden a few weeks to come. At the spinal cord, a protective substance referred to as myelin starts to wrap around it and the umbilical cord grows longer and stronger. The fetus' heartbeat is controlled by its brain and is now at 140 to 150 beats per minute, (twice as fast as how it will be at birth). Weeks to come, the pads in the toes and fingertips should be adorned with fingerprints. Sweat glands are now forming all over the body.

Body changes

At this time, you might be experiencing increased sensitivities to allergens and have probably noted a slight vaginal discharge. This is normal. It is also a common thing to develop a snoring habit due to stuffing in the nose but that can be solved by sleeping on a number of pillows to keep the head slightly elevated. What might be a bother though is increased appetite that doesn't go easily even with a whole tray of baked ziti or a three-pound lobster serving with lots of butter! Regardless of the surging craving, ensure that you don't follow the concept of eating for two to help control weight gain.

Week 18

This week, the fetus' bones will ossify or become harder, especially the feet and the inner ears, as its hearing become sharper. Furthermore, a few teeth and the blood vessels are fully developed and can be visible under the translucent skin. If your fetus is a girl, its uterus and fallopian tubes will fully develop in their correct positions. And although the growth rate of the fetus may tend to slow down, body movements such as somersaults and bending limb and joints remain persistent.

Your body changes

It's highly likely that you'll experience a sharp pain and aches in regions such as legs, tailbone and other muscles due to the fetus' rapid and frequent movements. And as the pregnancy hormones work on joints and ligaments, you might also experience headaches and back pains. You are also likely to be anxious or worried about whether the pregnancy is alright. Simply talk to a midwife or doctor if anxiety takes over your emotional life.

Week 19

The fetus weighs half a pound and measures about 6 inches. Despite having a bigger head, the arms and legs are proportional to the body and the fetus can manage all limb movements. The entire skin being covered with fine hair and creamy material called vernix caseosa that serves to protect the scalp. The greasy protective material is comprised of materials such as dead skin cells, oils from oils glands and the old lanugo. The hair on the scalp might also start to sprout although this varies in different unborn babies.

Your body changes

You might experience various skin changes and blotchy patches in areas such as nose, cheek, forehead and the chin. The skin might turn dry and flaky whereby you develop rashes on those stretched skin parts. If you have this problem, drinking a lot of water can help hydrate the skin, while oils and lotions can fight itching and dryness. Other mums may experience leg cramps that radiate up and down the calves particularly during the day. Such spasms could be brought about by fatigue brought by the weight of pregnancy. You can treat leg cramps by straightening the leg and then carefully flexing the ankle and toes back towards the shins.

Dietary tips

In order to support the brain cells of the fetus, ensure to eat healthy sources of fats like avocadoes, olive oils and fish. That's not all; ensure that 25-30 percent of your calories come from healthy fats as these form building blocks for the fetal cells. Also, eat fortified grain foods, lentils, dark leafy green veggies and fruits like oranges and melon to prevent possible birth defects.

Week 20

At 9-11 ounces, the digestive system of the fetus is fully working and should soon excrete a dark green sticky substance referred to as meconium. This waste substance is processed from amniotic fluid and cell loss initially swallowed with digestive secretions. By now, the sex organs like uterus and testicles are fully developed and an ultrasound scan can clearly tell the gender of the fetus. As the fetus can detect and respond to various stimuli, you should consider relaxing in quiet environments to allow the unborn baby to sleep for about 20 hours per day.

Your body changes

If you haven't felt any baby kicks by now, don't worry as it usually happens between week 18 and 22. Actually, thinner women are more likely to experience baby kicks earlier as opposed to those with thicker tissues. Nonetheless, this week, the uterus should get in line with your belly button; and it begins to grow to the direction of the rib cage at a rate of centimeter per week. Your nails might grow stronger and the hair tends to grow faster, fuller and thicker. The change is brought about by hormones and increased circulation that ensures hair and nails get required nutrients for quicker growth.

Week 21

Weighing around 11 pounds and 7 inches long, the fetus' umbilical cord continues to grow and thicken in order to facilitate supply of nutrients, blood and air. The fetus can by now differentiate flavors in amniotic fluids thanks to the developing taste buds. The eyebrows and the eyelids have also become fully developed. Fingernails and toenails also become fully developed.

The fetus' body is still covered with the soft hair referred to as lanugo to help regulate body temperatures.

Your body changes

At this point, you are highly likely to develop varicose veins in areas such as legs because of the uterus exerting pressure on inferior vena cava. You could also develop pink, red and purple stretch marks in areas like breasts, hips, belly and butt due to rapid growth of breasts and the belly. But despite the stretch marks, it's highly likely that you will feel better and more energized and if so, do some exercises.

Week 22

The physical size of the fetus resembles a spaghetti squash but might appear slightly thinner due to absence of fatty tissues. Although the eyes are fully formed, the colored part of the eye, known as the iris, still lacks pigment and is colorless. Despite this, the fetus has a complete sensory system and thus can "learn a few things" through touching or by rubbing against the uterine wall.

The liver is still able to secrete enzymes required to generate red blood cells such as bilirubin enzyme. Furthermore, the fetus can differentiate between light and darkness and can recognize your heartbeat or blood circulation in the body. In case the unborn you are expecting is a girl, the egg cells, uterus, and ovaries should be fully formed by the end of the week.

Your body changes

A more serious problem to be worried about is frequent vaginal discharge and possible yeast infections as a result of the dump environment. It is important to get your iron levels checked due to loss of iron through vaginal discharge, which can lead to anemia or trigger hemorrhage at the time of delivery.

Around this time, the uterus rises about 1 1/2 to 2 inches above the belly button, and the baby bump is clearly visible. But even though the belly has grown twice or thrice as bigger, this shouldn't prevent you from bending down, sitting or driving.

Week 23

From this week henceforth, the fetus begins to put on considerable weight and although for now weighs slightly over a pound, this weight should double in the next 4-weeks. The rapid change in weight is attributed to development of fat deposits under the skin, which should straighten the saggy skin in due time. The fetus also starts to take shape and should appear as a "small doll" on an ultrasound scanner! However, the skin may still appear loose or saggy due to a more rapid production of skin tissues compared to the fat layer. Another notable development is a red skin pigment, which is caused by growth of veins and arteries under the skin. If your fetus would be a baby boy, the testicles should start to descend into the groin area.

Your body changes

In addition to the varicose veins, the feet and ankles are likely to swell because of a condition referred to as edema, which causes the blood to be returned to the lower half of the body. A related problem can be the formation of red pigmentation on the soles of your feet and palms of your hands, which can make you to become extremely reactive to skin tags and heat rush. Other women also experience a skin discoloration around the eyes, nose, cheeks and forehead but such signs are temporary and go away in a few weeks.

As the fetus gains weight, you should have gained around 15 pounds by now. To prevent any complications, it is important to have a healthcare officer monitor your weight and the expanding uterus.

Week 24

The fetus weight has increased to about 1 ½ pounds and now measures 9-12 inches in length. The fetus respiratory system is working and has various cells that facilitate the lungs to both inflate and deflate. This lung movement is facilitated by production of surfactant, a substance that helps inflate air sacs in the lung when the fetus breathes in and out. Lack of surfactant can lead to premature birth or cause the baby to develop major defects in the respiratory system. As no air is available in the uterus, the fetus continues to inhale amniotic fluid, which is used to breathing practices. The fetus is also using hands and feet to touch and moves across the uterus and can cause hiccups or spasms in the diaphragm.

Your body changes

Due to increase in the size of the uterus, the belly button pops up resulting to pain and numbness in areas such as fingers, hands and wrists. Your navel protrudes as the uterus continues to swell and push the abdomen forward. Moreover, you're likely to feel tired and dizzy and or develop occasional heart burn. The dizziness is mostly caused by low blood sugar and is often triggered when you stand too fast. Therefore, you should learn to eat regularly and rise slowly if need be. But if you feel dizzy all the times, or feel like fainting, contact/visit your OB or doctor, as this might be a sign of anemia.

Week 25

The fetus weighs slightly over 1 ½ pounds and is now appearing plumper because of continued fat deposit under the skin. The skin has also softened a bit and the hair has a pigment and a good looking texture. As the lungs produce surfactant, the nostrils that had been clogged begin to open and the fetus can freely breathe in amniotic fluid. At this stage, baby movements tend to go overboard such that you could be worried that the fetus is hyperactive. However, this is nothing to worry about. You can press your partner's ear against your uterus to enable him to hear the fetus' heartbeat.

Your body changes

A rather common problem is back and hip pains but these can be relieved through walking, yoga, swimming and other non-weight-bearing exercises. Apart from usual pregnancy symptoms like dizziness, fatigue and occasional back pains, you might develop a serious case of hemorrhoids. This condition is characterized by swollen veins around the rectum due to increased blood supply to the rectum. Hemorrhoids are uncomfortable and painful and can in some cases cause rectal bleeding or worsen underlying constipation problems.

Week 26

The fetus weight has doubled to 2 pounds and has grown in length to about 14 inches. The eyelids that had remained shut so far begin to open and the fetus can perceive a flashlight placed near the uterus. As its eyesight improves, the peripheral sensory end organs and cochlea (part of the ear) continue to develop and this causes increased activity in response to stimuli. By now, the heart of the fetus can pump blood, the lungs have fully developed blood vessels and the circulatory system is now fully functional. Although the fetus may still appear lean, there's continuous accumulation of body fat that should continue until delivery.

Your body changes

Common pregnancy symptoms that were present in the first trimester like frequent urination and fatigue are common during this period. This is coupled with leg cramps, sleeplessness and heartburn. You might also find it harder to sleep on the back since the pregnancy may work against your backbone and cut off blood flow.

Week 27

The fetus weighs about 2 ¼ pounds and should begin to curl face down in the uterus in what is referred to as "fetal position". This week, the eyes continue to form particularly the retina layers and eyelids, which mean that the fetus can now open and close eyes properly. Baby movements are common than ever before since the fetus responds to sounds, light flashes and other stimuli with hiccupping. Most fetuses should have developed a particular sleeping and waking up pattern and this helps control constant movements. It is important to ensure that the baby gets maximum rest during sleeping period.

Your body changes

With the third trimester approaching, the uterus has significantly increased in size and it's practically impossible to hide the pregnancy. Moreover, the increase in fetus size causes the volume of the amniotic fluid to reduce to almost by half. In some cases, you might note the elbows and bony knees of the unborn baby poke out of the belly! On the bad side, you might experience tingling pains in your legs and lower back, which may make bending down or walking very painful. Your hands, feet and ankles may also continue to swell because of increased bodily fluids.

Pregnancy Tips For Second Semester

1. Whenever You Feel Like Working Out, These Exercising Tips Can Help A Lot

-Walk on a treadmill or take <u>long walks</u> outdoors to safely build up endurance for labor. Here, you can do some sitting cycling at least 20 times for each leg in a day.

-You can also try some <u>kegel exercises</u> to help tone up pelvic floor muscles and the uterus. Sit on a chair or bed and squeeze your pelvic floor muscles by contracting inwards tightly and holding for some seconds. A simpler way is to picture yourself peeing then hold and release repeatedly.

-Do squats with a chair to maintain your balance. Put your legs apart and lower yourself by bending the knees. As you do this, stick your bottom out and then lean forward at the waist.

-Do some 'tummy sucking" technique. Just pretend to inhale with your stomach. Then exhale by relaxing your abdominal muscles to pull your belly toward your belly button. Repeat this technique a couple of times.

2. If Finding Harder To Sleep Due To Baby Movements And Other Pains, Try Out These Tips:

-Sleep on the left side of your belly, as it's more accommodating for your growing belly. At 16 weeks and beyond, sleeping on your back causes the fetus to press on your blood vessels. To sleep well, lie on your left side with the knees up, preferably with 2 or more pillows placed between the knees to increase comfort. If you often roll on your back, use pillows to help maintain you on the left side. Sleeping on the left side also keeps the pressure off the muscles around the pelvis and hips.

-Create a bed-time routine where you sleep and wake up at regular times. If you have a long lie-in say in the morning, you might find it harder to fall asleep at night.

-Find time to relax a few hours before bedtime. In this case, you shouldn't do strenuous exercises or watch TV for long to avoid unnecessary fatigue or stress. Instead, have a bath, read a book, meditate, or drink a warm milky drink. Repeat the pattern 1-2 hours before you sleep.

3. Dietary Tips

Be aware that in the second trimester, you are eating for two; therefore, you must eat at least 2000-2500 calories each day. Follow these tips:

-To boost protein intake, consume meat such as fish, pork, poultry, baked beans, canned fish, chicken thighs and ground beef. If you don't like meat, peas and lentils are good alternatives as they are also rich in proteins.

-Increase your vegetables and fruits intake to get the vitamins and minerals required to support the pregnancy. Veggies are good sources of magnesium, fiber, iron, vitamins A and vitamin C so ensure that you eat 4 to 5 servings of vegetables daily and 4 servings of fruits daily. Go for some squash, turnip, potatoes, unsweetened fruit packed juice, cabbage, macaroni, fried bread, carrots, barley, rolled oats and apples.

-Eat three servings of dairy products a day such as milk, yoghurt and cheese. They are good sources of phosphorous, calcium, protein, vitamin B, proteins, iron and zinc.

-Eat 10 servings in a day of whole-grains and fortified foods as they will energize you and supply your unborn baby with the needed nutrients for growth. Foods such as cereals, bread, rice and pasta are good for your health at this stage. These foods have folic acid and iron too, which help prevent diseases like anemia.

Third Trimester

Week 28

In this first week of your third trimester, your baby is about 16 inches long and weighs about 2 ½ pounds. Looking at ultrasound image of your baby, you can note the plump appearance due to fat deposits under the skin. At this stage, the eyes are totally opened with the eyelids and eyebrows fully formed. Moreover, eyelashes may now be visible. The enzyme production and endocrine glands continue to develop. The endocrine system helps the fetus produce internal secretions (hormones in particular) that are transported throughout the body by the bloodstream. The fetus should start to shift into head down pose anytime from now towards delivery.

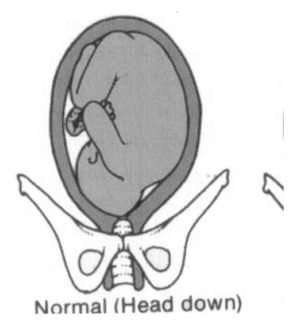

Normal (Head down)

Your body changes

The belly has grown bigger and bigger and you may no longer feel comfortable doing basic tasks like bending or exercising. You might also experience sharp pain in your lower spine as the fetus' head rests on the sciatic nerve. The sharp tingling pain is caused by the fetus shifting into "fetus position" and can be extreme in some cases.

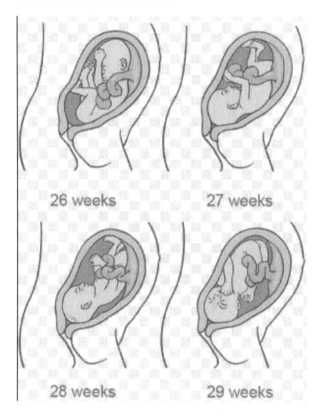

26 weeks   27 weeks

28 weeks   29 weeks

Week 29

The fetus measures 16-inches in length and weighs 3 pounds. The fetus' teeth buds start to develop permanent teeth on the gums, while the Androgens start to produce an estrogen-like chemical that helps in your milk production. The chemical is converted into estriol by the placenta and triggers your body to start producing milk to breastfed the baby after delivery. For a couple of weeks now, your baby's kicks will go overboard and probably cause severe rib pain or pelvic pains. However, as the baby continues to grow, the hyperactivity decreases as most of the room is occupied in the uterus.

Your body changes

As the fetus continues to kick, this can cause unintentional loss of urine, which can be somehow uncomfortable. Furthermore, your breasts also start to secrete a milky substance called colostrum that may often dampen your bra often. Then, you might experience increased hunger as your baby utilizes most of your nutrients; you have to eat frequently but in small amounts. At this time, varicose veins, hemorrhoids and purplish-red spider veins are persistent due to increased blood flow.

Week 30

The fetus is now 2 months from delivery but may still appear wrinkled due to irregular fat distribution on its body. However, as fat deposits continue to build, wrinkles on the skin will smoothen out, although the hair cover, called lanugo, still persists on the skin. Soon, the lanugo will disappear as the fetus comes into full maturity. This week, the fetus' brain acquires grooves and indentations, which facilitate increase in brain tissue and sensory responses.

Your body changes

You might experience flutters within the uterus as the fetus hiccups while practicing breathing, and moves its diaphragm up and down. Furthermore, you could experience shortness of breath since the uterus presses hard on your diaphragm. At other times, you should experience frequent urination problems, indigestion and heartburn. The main cause for heartburn is when food and digestive juices head upstream into your esophagus especially due to the increased pressure from below (because of the belly).

Week 31

The fetus weighs about 3-3.5 pounds and could measure anywhere between 15-18 inches. At this point, the fetus' lungs can now inflate fully due to the adequate amounts of surfactant, a substance that helps to inhibit possible collapse of the lungs after delivery. As the ears are fully developed, the fetus can now listen and respond to sounds and other stimuli, which demands that you avoid noisy areas. On average, the fetus can make ten kicks an hour and this should help determine its health or any defects before birth. It should also swallow and excrete amniotic fluid to sustain the digestive system running and curb possible gastrointestinal problems.

Your body changes

The most common problem at this stage is pains as the uterus begins to tighten and contract in preparation for delivery. Such an experience, referred to as *Braxton Hicks contractions*, could occur anytime from now but are normal and shouldn't cause unnecessary anxiety. As stated before, the problem of breathlessness may still persist as the uterus pushes the lungs and prevents free expansion. However, the unborn baby breathes through the placenta and is not in any danger.

Week 32

The fetus is rapidly gaining weight and by now weighs 4 pounds or more. As it grows in size, most of the uterine cavity is occupied and this could reduce hyperactivity. For now, the umbilical cord is coated with gelatinous substance that inhibits knots and kinks during twists and turns of your baby. Its skeleton is now fully formed although the bones particularly on the skull are soft and flexible to facilitate childbirth. In most cases, fetuses normally have their head-down or completely turned around position by now. Although this might take longer, failure to achieve the head-down position may suggest that delivery will happen through C-section.

Your body changes

The *Braxton Hicks Contractions* might take a toll on you and can, at high intensity, be very painful. These contractions basically occur for about 30 seconds and are characterized by tightening at the top of the uterus. Although they can seem to be like real labor, the contractions should not last beyond one minute. Another issue to be worried about is weight gain that basically comes from fluid retention or additional weight from the unborn baby.

Week 33

The fetus should measure between 17-19 inches and weighs around 4.5 pounds. The brain continues to grow and this may cause noticeable increase in the size of its head. The immune system is almost fully developed but would require at least 2 more weeks to mature up. With time, the amniotic fluid starts getting depleted and thinner and thus the fetus should easily differentiate days and nights. As the fetus grows to maturity, you should notice more breathing exercises and longer duration of sleeping.

Your body changes

From this week henceforth, you might feel better as kicking or baby movements are beginning to get scarce. But you need to take rest most of the times due to weight gain accompanied by persistent fatigue. If tiredness or insomnia makes it harder for you to relax, do not eat or exercise 1-2 hours before sleeping.

Week 34

At 5 pounds and measuring at least 18 inches, the fetus has almost matured and should be delivered anytime from week 38. Although all parts are fully developed, the lungs may still require a week or so to be ready for breathing. Moreover, the fetus should become plump, as more fat deposits accumulate on the skin, and those chubby cheeks probably might change its facial appearance! By now, the testicles in males should have descended into the scrotum and female sex organs mature too.

Your body changes

Right now, you won't experience major body changes. However, you may notice that you are becoming farsighted or nearsighted due to fluid retention around your eyes. Hormones can also inhibit tear production, which in turn make eyes dry and irritated. Nonetheless, keep in mind that blurry vision may not happen to everyone and is temporary.

Week 35

This week, the fetus should weigh almost 6 pounds and measure around 18 inches. As the fat deposits are more evident, the hair covering called lanugo has greatly reduced and finer hair called vellus starts to replace them. The amniotic fluid is getting thinner but the skull remains soft to facilitate the baby to pass easily in your birth canal.

Your body changes

The usual problem of frequent urination may haunt you again this time because of the fetus adopting the face down position. Such a pose presses hard on your bladder and can trigger unintentional urination when you cough or sneeze. By now, the enlarged uterus that is beyond 10 times its normal volume makes it harder to change positions or breathe easily.

Week 36

Almost 9 months down the line, your unborn baby is reaching fully maturity and is about 19 inches in length and weighing around 6 pounds. Although birth dates vary from woman to woman and from pregnancy to pregnancy, you are now about one week or so to giving birth. The unborn being is now considered a baby (not a fetus), and continues to accumulate fat deposits under the skin, which may cause the arms, legs, cheeks, knees and face to appear plumpish. After delivery, the digestive system and lungs should begin to function on their own but for now, the baby relies on the umbilical cord.

Your body changes

By now, you should be preparing for labor and thus it is usual to experience pelvic pains as the baby presses the head against the pelvis. However, with time, the baby should drop from the uterus right into the pelvic cavity, and this can help you feel better. If you find pelvic pains too much to bear, try getting warm compresses, massages or warm baths preferably from your midwife.

Week 37

The growth rate for your baby is greatly reduced to around 0.5 ounces in day. The head that had been too large should now attain the same circumference as the other body parts to facilitate delivery. And the lanugo hair should have disappeared alongside other protective substances like the vernix caseosa. The hair is also growing rapidly; and depending on the baby's genetics, the scalp may be full of hair. Most babies should weigh between 6-7 pounds by delivery time.

Your body changes

You might not experience any new changes apart from slight increase in vaginal discharge that comprise of mucus-like substance. This is referred to as cervical mucus plug and it helps prepare you for the forthcoming labor, i.e. to facilitate easier passage of the baby during delivery. At this stage, it is advisable to visit your doctor to check if the cervix has opened enough before you get into labor.

Week 38

This week, the baby is head-down position on your pelvic bone, and it's also likely that you give birth as well. But if you haven't given birth by now, the baby continues to grow. It may grow up to 21 inches in length and weigh over 7 pounds. In preparation for neonate's initial cry, the tear ducts are forming and your baby should now be clenching fists awaiting delivery. Any remaining lanugo and vernix is shed into the amniotic fluid and eventually eaten by the baby. When excreted, the waste product forms the first bowel movement referred to as meconium.

Your body changes

A common phenomenon is to experience "leaky breast" in which your breasts release a yellowish liquid referred to as colostrum. If this is a bother, it's advisable to fit nursing pads inside your bra until everything gets back to normal. By now, the cervix is likely to have dilated to facilitate child birth that should occur as soon as now!

Week 39

The pregnancy is now at full term, but if delivery doesn't take place, the baby may continue to grow but with decrease in levels of amniotic fluid. The unborn baby may continue to produce surfactant to help prevent the lung sacs from sticking to each other during initial breathing. Although the tear ducts are now fully formed, they aren't open yet so the baby might not shed tears right at birth.

Your body changes

Here you should be expecting the earliest signs for labor such as the rupture of the amniotic sac to release the amniotic fluid. Also, be aware of bloody discharge after capillaries rupture at the cervix, diarrhea, nausea and the loss of mucus plug at the cervix. If you don't notice any blood or signs of delivery, you may consider visiting a health officer so as to check the condition of your pregnancy.

Week 40

Your baby is awaiting delivery and may not be growing any further. Actually, organs such as the brain and lungs are expected to develop further after childbirth, so everything is okay now. The baby has also developed immunity needed to fight possible infections after birth. In cases of delayed pregnancy, the unborn baby may grow up to 22 inches in length while weighing up to 10 pounds. The skull bones should have separated so that they can effortlessly pass through your birth canal.

Your body changes

Labor pains may now be approaching, a sign that you are now at delivery. However, if you have not yet have delivered, your pregnancy is considered post-term. Meanwhile, take notice of any yellowish fluid from your birth canal as this could signify rupture of the amniotic fluid. If nothing changes from now hence forth, consider calling your doctor to inspect your cervix or conduct other relevant tests.

Beyond week 40

Strange as it may sound, you might carry the pregnancy up to 2 weeks from now. However, don't take chances before you're aware of the condition of the pregnancy. Talking to a doctor may help you learn possible methods of speeding up labor and delivery.

Pregnancy Tips for Third Semester

1. Dealing with pregnancy changes in this semester

Common problems in third trimester include as backaches, bleeding, fatigue, frequent urination, heartburn and constipation. Other short-term problems may include hemorrhoids, spider and varicose veins and weight gain. However, you should contact a doctor for severe symptoms like serious bleeding, severe dizziness, pain or burning during urination, severe vomiting, abdominal cramps and rapid weight change.

Let's see how you can manage some of these issues:

-If you experience shortness of breath, try propping your head and shoulders up with pillows during sleep.

-For Braxton hick's contractions, talk to your mid-wife or doctor especially if such contractions are making you to have shortness of breath or are attacking you regularly.

-If you note sudden rush of fluid or if the vaginal discharge is heavy enough to soak your inner wears, call your doctor immediately.

-Persistent swelling: unusual or sudden swelling could be a sign of preeclampsia, a risky condition that demands medical attention. Call your doctor.

2. Follow proper nutrition

-Ensure that you consume at least 2400 calories daily; spread this up into small regular meals and snacks. Ensure that you chew food well to facilitate an easy digestion and maximum absorption.

-To avoid heartburn, don't lie down after eating to avoid acid refluxing back into the esophagus. To make this work, try to raise your head and shoulders when eating and eat less greasy foods. If necessary, take lots of warm fresh water in between meals but not with meals because this could make the problem worse. Also, ditch drinks such as coffee, soda, alcohol and tobacco.

3. Exercising techniques

Exercising on the third trimester could be a nightmare due to additional weight and bigger belly but ensure you do simple exercises like walking along with other simple home chores. However, alternate exercise with enough rest to help both you and your baby relax. That said, only do exercises that focus on joint mobility, flexibility and labor preparation such as butterfly stretches and stretch poses. Let's see how to get started:

✓ Sleeping stretch pose

-Lie on your back and interlock the fingers of both hands beneath the head

-Then bend your knees keeping the soles of your feet on the floor

-Then tilt your head in the opposite direction and repeat severally.

✓ Butterfly Stretch

-Stretch your legs out, then bend the right leg and then place the right foot on the left thigh as far as you can.

-Put the right hand right on top of the right knee (bent).

-Then proceed to hold the toes of the right foot with the left hand.

- Gently move your right knee up towards your chest while you breathe in gently.

4. Prepare for Labor beforehand

- Attend classes with your partner to learn techniques of handling pain such as visualization stretches that strengthen the muscles surrounding your uterus.

- Decide whether to go to the hospital or if you'd love to deliver at home through your midwife.

- Obtain the day and night phone contacts of your medics just in case your water breaks suddenly or at unexpected times.

- Cater for transportation especially if you stay alone; and arrange for shopping supplies for your newborn's necessities. A mid-wife should help you on this.

Breaking of Water

When that moment comes when water breaks, you experience a sensation of wetness within your vagina, continuous trickling of small amounts of some watery fluid from your vagina, wetness of your perineum or an obvious gush of water (like they do in movies!), don't panic. Before you do anything, keep in mind that you shouldn't do anything that could end up introducing bacterial into your vagina (including taking a bath!); just visit your doctor. If you are not sure whether it is urine or amniotic fluid (because you experience a feeling of wetness or just a trickle of fluid), visit your doctor if you are due. They will confirm it for you. Read more about labor <u>here</u>.

Conclusion

Thank you again for downloading this book!

I hope this book was able to help you to understand how everything about your baby as he/she develops. Congratulations!

The next step is to use this information.

Thank you and good luck!

Preview Of - Pregnancy: Expecting A Baby For New Moms

This book gives you a comprehensive understanding of how your baby is developing week for week as well as what it is you should do to ensure you have a healthy and successful pregnancy.

When that home pregnancy test kit or blood test returns positive, your world spines off. Immediately, you start thinking of all the things you out to buy, all the ways you ought to prepare, and all the changes you will undergo.

Amidst the excitement, it is normal to feel panicky because the thought of carrying a baby to term, taking care of your health as well as the health of the baby and caring for a baby after birth is overwhelming.

The best way to prepare yourself for motherhood as well as pregnancy is to become knowledgeable. In this guide, **Expecting a Baby for New Moms**, we shall look at, and understand the trimesters and the changes you can expect to see as your pregnancy progresses. You will also learn about how to take care of your health and your baby's as well as how to prepare for labor and child birth.

Enjoying Reading My Books? Maybe You Want To Read These Books Too

Below you'll find some of my other books that are on Amazon and Kindle as well. Simply click on the links below to check them out.

Want to know when next book is released? Subscribe here: www.lacobiz.com

Pregnancy: Expecting A Baby For New Moms

Recommended:

Ketogenic Diet: Top 50 Breakfast Recipes

Ketogenic Diet: Top 50 Lunch Recipes

Ketogenic Diet: Top 50 Dinner Recipes

Yoga: Beginners Guide - For Yoga Poses - Easy Steps And Pictures

Mindfulness - Meditation For Beginners – Stress Free Body, Depression And Anxiety Relief

5 Weeks Ketogenic Plan, Weight Loss Recipes - Easy Steps For beginners

Ketogenic: Ketogenic Diet - Mistakes Protection Handbook

Smoothies Cleanse - Detox Diet And Lose Weight In A Healthy Way

Don't forget to subscribe to my newsletter! www.lacobiz.com

Made in the USA
Columbia, SC
29 May 2018